SLEEPLESS YOUTH

Understanding and Overcoming Teenage Sleep Deprivation

Dr. Christine Peters

About Author

Dr. Christine Peters is a mental health professional known for her contributions to the field of psychology. Her work often focuses on clinical practice, therapeutic techniques, and mental health research.

Dr. Peters has been involved in developing and promoting evidence-based treatments and interventions for various mental health conditions. She may also engage in writing and speaking engagements to further educate both professionals and the public about mental health issues and advancements in the field.

Table of Contents

Chapter 1. Introduction to Insomnia

Understanding the Basics

Insomnia, often regarded as the most common sleep disorder, affects millions of people worldwide. It is characterized by difficulty falling asleep, staying asleep, or waking up too early and being unable to return to sleep. Unlike occasional sleeplessness, which everyone experiences from time to time, insomnia is a persistent problem that can significantly impact one's daily life and overall well-being.

The causes of insomnia are varied and multifaceted, ranging from psychological factors like stress and anxiety to physical issues such as chronic pain or respiratory problems. Environmental factors, including noise, light, and uncomfortable temperatures, can also contribute to sleep disturbances. Additionally, lifestyle choices, such as irregular sleep schedules, excessive caffeine or alcohol consumption, and lack of physical activity, play a crucial role in the development and maintenance of insomnia.

Insomnia can be classified into two main types: acute and chronic. Acute insomnia is short-term and often linked to specific stressors or changes in routine. It usually resolves on its own once the stressor is removed or the individual adapts to the change. Chronic insomnia, on the other hand, persists for at least three nights per week for three months or longer and often requires a comprehensive treatment approach.

The Importance of Sleep

Sleep is a fundamental biological need, as essential to survival as food and water. It is a complex process that involves various stages, each playing a critical role in maintaining physical and mental health. During sleep, the body undergoes numerous restorative functions, including muscle growth, tissue repair, protein synthesis, and the release of growth hormones. Additionally, the brain processes and consolidates memories, clears out toxins, and regulates emotions, all of which are vital for cognitive function and emotional stability.

The repercussions of inadequate sleep are profound and far-reaching. In the short term, sleep deprivation can lead to impaired concentration, memory lapses, and decreased performance at work or school. It also increases the risk of accidents and injuries, as alertness and reaction times are compromised. Long-term sleep deprivation is associated with a host of serious health problems, including cardiovascular disease, diabetes, obesity, and weakened immune function. It also exacerbates mental health issues such as depression and anxiety, creating a vicious cycle that further disrupts sleep.

Understanding the importance of sleep underscores the necessity of addressing insomnia effectively. Quality sleep is not a luxury but a cornerstone of health and well-being. By prioritizing sleep and implementing proven strategies to combat insomnia, individuals can improve their quality of life, enhance productivity, and safeguard their physical and mental health.

In conclusion, insomnia is a pervasive and debilitating condition that demands attention and action. Recognizing its causes and understanding the critical importance of sleep are the first steps toward finding a solution. This book will explore a range of strategies and treatments to help readers reclaim their nights and achieve the restful, restorative sleep they deserve.

Chapter 2. The Science of Sleep

Sleep Stages and Cycles

Sleep is a complex and dynamic process that involves multiple stages and cycles, each playing a critical role in maintaining overall health and well-being. Understanding these stages and how they work can shed light on the mechanisms of sleep and the impact of sleep disorders like insomnia.

Stages of Sleep

Sleep is broadly divided into two types: Rapid Eye Movement (REM) sleep and Non-Rapid Eye Movement (NREM) sleep. NREM sleep is further subdivided into three stages:

1. **Stage N1 (NREM 1):** This is the lightest stage of sleep, lasting only a few minutes. During this stage, the body begins to relax,

and brain activity slows. People can be easily awakened in N1, often experiencing hypnic jerks or the sensation of falling.

2. **Stage N2 (NREM 2):** This stage represents a deeper level of sleep, where heart rate and body temperature drop. Brain activity shows distinct patterns known as sleep spindles and K-complexes, which are thought to protect sleep and assist in memory consolidation. N2 sleep accounts for about 50% of the total sleep cycle.

3. **Stage N3 (NREM 3):** Also known as slow-wave sleep (SWS) or deep sleep, this stage is crucial for physical restoration and recovery. During N3, the brain produces slow delta waves, and waking someone up

from this stage is difficult. Deep sleep plays a significant role in repairing tissues, building muscle, and strengthening the immune system.

REM Sleep

After progressing through the NREM stages, the body enters REM sleep. REM sleep is characterized by rapid eye movements, increased brain activity, and vivid dreams. It is essential for cognitive functions, including learning, memory consolidation, and emotional regulation. During REM sleep, the body undergoes atonia, a temporary paralysis of most voluntary muscles, which prevents individuals from acting out their dreams. REM sleep cycles typically occur every 90 minutes and increase in duration as the night progresses.

Sleep Cycles

A full sleep cycle, including both NREM and REM sleep, lasts about 90 to 110 minutes. Throughout the night, individuals typically experience four to six sleep cycles. The composition of these cycles changes, with deep sleep (N3) dominating the early part of the night and REM sleep increasing in the latter part. Understanding these cycles is vital for appreciating how disruptions, such as those caused by insomnia, can impact overall sleep quality and health.

The Role of Circadian Rhythms

Circadian rhythms are natural, internal processes that regulate the sleep-wake cycle and repeat roughly every 24 hours. These rhythms are driven by the brain's biological clock, located in the suprachiasmatic nucleus (SCN) of the hypothalamus. Circadian rhythms are influenced by external cues, known as zeitgebers, with light being the most powerful.

Biological Clock and Melatonin

The SCN responds to light and dark signals received through the eyes. In the presence of light, the SCN inhibits the production of melatonin, a hormone that promotes sleep, keeping us awake and alert during the day. As night falls and light diminishes, the SCN signals the pineal gland to release melatonin, preparing the body for sleep.

Circadian Disruptions

Disruptions to circadian rhythms can have profound effects on sleep and overall health. Common disruptions include shift work, jet lag, and exposure to artificial light at night. These disruptions can lead to difficulties in falling asleep, staying asleep, and obtaining restorative sleep, contributing to conditions like insomnia.

Chronotypes

People have different chronotypes, which are natural preferences for sleeping and waking times. Morning chronotypes (early birds) tend to wake up early and feel more alert in the morning, while evening chronotypes (night owls) prefer to stay up late and wake up later. Understanding one's chronotype can help optimize sleep patterns and improve sleep quality.

The science of sleep encompasses the intricate stages and cycles of sleep and the critical role of circadian rhythms in regulating the sleep-wake cycle. By understanding these processes, we can better appreciate the complexities of sleep and the importance of maintaining a regular sleep schedule to combat insomnia and enhance overall health.

Chapter 3. Common Causes of Insomnia

Stress and Anxiety

Stress and anxiety are among the most prevalent causes of insomnia. When faced with stressful situations, the body's natural response is to release stress hormones like cortisol and adrenaline. These hormones prepare the body for a "fight or flight" response, increasing alertness and making it difficult to relax and fall asleep. While this response is useful in short-term emergencies, chronic stress can lead to prolonged sleep difficulties.

Impact of Stress on Sleep

Stress triggers a cascade of physiological and psychological reactions that can severely disrupt sleep. Elevated cortisol levels can interfere with the ability to fall asleep and stay asleep, leading to fragmented sleep and reduced time spent in restorative deep and REM sleep stages. Additionally, stress often leads to racing thoughts and excessive worrying, which can keep the mind active and prevent the onset of sleep.

Anxiety Disorders and Sleep

Anxiety disorders, including generalized anxiety disorder (GAD), panic disorder, and post-traumatic stress disorder (PTSD), are closely linked with insomnia. People with these conditions often experience heightened arousal and hypervigilance, making it challenging to achieve the calm state necessary for sleep. The anticipation of not being able to sleep can itself become a source of anxiety, perpetuating a vicious cycle of sleeplessness.

Coping Mechanisms

Addressing stress and anxiety is crucial for improving sleep. Techniques such as cognitive behavioral therapy for insomnia (CBT-I), mindfulness meditation, and relaxation exercises can help manage stress and reduce anxiety, promoting better sleep. Establishing a bedtime routine that includes calming activities like reading, taking a warm bath, or practicing deep breathing can also signal to the body that it's time to wind down.

Lifestyle and Environmental Factors

Lifestyle choices and environmental factors play a significant role in the onset and persistence of insomnia. Our daily habits and surroundings can either support or hinder our ability to get quality sleep.

Lifestyle Factors

1. **Irregular Sleep Schedules:** Keeping inconsistent sleep and wake times can disrupt the body's internal clock, making it harder to maintain a regular sleep pattern. This is common among shift workers, travelers, and individuals with erratic schedules.

2. **Diet and Caffeine Consumption:** Consuming large meals, caffeine, or alcohol

close to bedtime can interfere with sleep. Caffeine is a stimulant that can keep the brain alert, while alcohol, although initially sedating, can disrupt sleep later in the night.

3. **Lack of Physical Activity:** Regular physical activity promotes better sleep, but a sedentary lifestyle can contribute to sleep difficulties. However, exercising too close to bedtime can have the opposite effect, as it raises body temperature and stimulates alertness.

4. **Excessive Screen Time:** Exposure to screens emitting blue light (from phones, tablets, computers, and TVs) before bedtime can interfere with melatonin production, delaying sleep onset. The stimulating

content and interactive nature of screens can also keep the mind engaged.

Environmental Factors

1. **Noise:** Environmental noise, whether from traffic, neighbors, or household appliances, can disrupt sleep. Sudden or continuous sounds can prevent individuals from falling asleep or wake them during the night.

2. **Light:** Exposure to artificial light, especially blue light, can trick the brain into thinking it's daytime, suppressing melatonin production and delaying sleep. Light pollution from streetlights or indoor lighting can also interfere with sleep.

3. **Temperature:** The sleep environment should be cool, quiet, and dark. Extremes in temperature—whether too hot or too cold—can make it difficult to fall asleep or stay asleep comfortably.

4. **Uncomfortable Bedding:** An uncomfortable mattress or pillow can cause physical discomfort and pain, leading to difficulty falling asleep and frequent awakenings. Investing in quality bedding that supports the body can make a significant difference in sleep quality.

Improving Sleep Hygiene

Adopting good sleep hygiene practices can mitigate the impact of lifestyle and environmental factors on sleep. This includes maintaining a consistent sleep schedule, creating a relaxing bedtime routine, limiting exposure to screens and bright lights before bed, ensuring the sleep environment is comfortable, and avoiding stimulants and large meals close to bedtime.

Understanding the common causes of insomnia—such as stress, anxiety, and various lifestyle and environmental factors—provides a foundation for addressing and overcoming sleep difficulties.

Chapter 4. Types of Insomnia

Acute vs. Chronic Insomnia

Acute Insomnia

Acute insomnia, also known as short-term insomnia, is a temporary sleep disturbance that typically lasts for a few days to a few weeks. It is often triggered by specific life events or stressors, such as a stressful work situation, a significant life change, or a temporary illness. Acute insomnia can also result from changes in routine, such as traveling across time zones or adjusting to a new work schedule.

Characteristics of Acute Insomnia:

- **Duration:** Lasts for a short period, typically less than three months.

- **Cause:** Often linked to identifiable stressors or changes in routine.

- **Resolution:** Usually resolves on its own once the triggering factors are removed or addressed.

Chronic Insomnia

Chronic insomnia is a more persistent condition, characterized by difficulty falling asleep or staying asleep at least three times per week for three months or longer. Unlike acute insomnia, chronic insomnia often involves an ongoing pattern of sleep disturbances that can be influenced by a range of factors, including underlying health conditions or long-standing stressors.

Characteristics of Chronic Insomnia:

- **Duration:** Lasts for three months or longer, with frequent disruptions in sleep.

- **Cause:** May involve multiple factors, including persistent stress, lifestyle issues, or underlying medical conditions.

- **Resolution:** Requires a more comprehensive approach to treatment and management, often involving lifestyle changes, therapy, and sometimes medication.

Primary and Secondary Insomnia

Primary Insomnia

Primary insomnia is defined as a sleep disorder that is not directly attributable to any other medical condition or external cause. It is characterized by difficulty initiating or maintaining sleep that is not better explained by other factors such as medication side effects, psychiatric disorders, or substance use.

Characteristics of Primary Insomnia:

- **No Identifiable Cause:** The insomnia itself is the primary issue, without any other underlying medical or psychiatric conditions directly contributing.

- **Diagnosis:** Typically diagnosed when sleep disturbances are not linked to other health conditions or external factors.

- **Treatment:** Often involves behavioral therapies, sleep hygiene improvements, and relaxation techniques to address the sleep issues directly.

Secondary Insomnia

Secondary insomnia, also known as comorbid insomnia, occurs as a result of another condition or factor. It is characterized by sleep disturbances that are secondary to other medical or psychiatric issues, such as chronic pain, depression, anxiety disorders, or substance abuse.

Characteristics of Secondary Insomnia:

- **Underlying Cause:** The insomnia is secondary to an underlying condition or factor, such as a health issue, medication side effect, or substance use.

- **Diagnosis:** Requires identification and treatment of the primary condition causing the sleep disturbances.

- **Treatment:** Focuses on managing the underlying condition in addition to addressing the insomnia, which may involve both medical treatment for the primary condition and behavioral interventions for the sleep disturbances.

Management Strategies:

- **For Primary Insomnia:** Strategies include cognitive behavioral therapy for insomnia (CBT-I), improvements in sleep hygiene, and relaxation techniques.

- **For Secondary Insomnia:** Treatment involves addressing the primary condition causing the insomnia, which may include medical management, psychotherapy, or lifestyle adjustments, alongside targeted interventions for sleep.

Recognizing the different types of insomnia—acute vs. chronic and primary vs. secondary—is essential for effective diagnosis and treatment. By identifying the nature and underlying causes of insomnia, individuals can tailor their approach to managing and overcoming sleep difficulties, improving overall sleep quality and well-being.

Chapter 5. Identifying Sleep Disorders

Sleep Apnea

Sleep apnea is a common sleep disorder characterized by repeated interruptions in breathing during sleep. These interruptions, known as apneas, can last for a few seconds to several minutes and occur numerous times throughout the night. Sleep apnea often leads to fragmented sleep, causing excessive daytime sleepiness and a range of health issues.

Types of Sleep Apnea:

1. **Obstructive Sleep Apnea (OSA):** The most common form, OSA occurs when the muscles in the throat relax excessively during sleep, leading to a blockage of the upper

airway. This obstruction results in reduced airflow and frequent awakenings to restore normal breathing.

2. **Central Sleep Apnea:** This less common type occurs when the brain fails to send the appropriate signals to the muscles that control breathing. Unlike OSA, central sleep apnea does not involve a physical blockage but rather a failure in the brain's respiratory control mechanisms.

3. **Complex Sleep Apnea Syndrome:** Also known as treatment-emergent central sleep apnea, this type is a combination of obstructive and central sleep apnea, often observed in individuals whose OSA does not fully resolve with treatment.

Symptoms of Sleep Apnea:

- Loud snoring

- Choking or gasping during sleep

- Excessive daytime sleepiness

- Difficulty concentrating or memory problems

- Morning headaches

- Dry mouth or sore throat upon waking

Diagnosis and Treatment:

Diagnosis typically involves a sleep study, either at home (home sleep apnea testing) or in a sleep clinic (polysomnography). Treatment options may include lifestyle changes (such as weight loss or positional therapy), the use of a continuous positive airway pressure (CPAP) machine to keep the airway open, or surgical interventions for severe cases.

Restless Leg Syndrome (RLS)

Restless Leg Syndrome (RLS), also known as Willis-Ekbom disease, is a neurological condition characterized by an uncontrollable urge to move the legs, often accompanied by uncomfortable sensations. These symptoms typically occur when at rest or during periods of inactivity, such as sitting or lying down, and are relieved by movement.

Symptoms of RLS:

- Unpleasant sensations in the legs, often described as crawling, tingling, or itching
- An overwhelming urge to move the legs to relieve discomfort

- Symptoms that worsen during periods of
  rest or inactivity

- Relief of symptoms through movement,
  such as walking or stretching

- Symptoms often occur in the evening or at
  night, potentially leading to difficulty falling
  or staying asleep

Diagnosis and Treatment:

Diagnosis is primarily based on clinical symptoms
and a detailed medical history. There is no specific
test for RLS, but ruling out other conditions and
evaluating iron levels through blood tests may be
part of the diagnostic process.

Treatment for RLS can involve lifestyle
modifications, such as improving sleep hygiene,

reducing caffeine and alcohol intake, and incorporating regular physical activity. In more severe cases, medical treatments may include medications that target dopamine imbalances, anticonvulsants, or iron supplements if deficiencies are identified.

Managing RLS:

- **Lifestyle Changes:** Regular exercise, maintaining a consistent sleep schedule, and avoiding triggers like caffeine can help manage symptoms.

- **Medical Therapies:** For persistent cases, medications like dopaminergic agents or iron supplements (for those with low iron levels) may be prescribed.

Identifying and understanding sleep disorders such as sleep apnea and Restless Leg Syndrome is crucial for effective management and treatment. Recognizing the symptoms and seeking appropriate medical evaluation can lead to targeted interventions, improving sleep quality and overall health.

Chapter 6. Cognitive Behavioral Therapy for Insomnia (CBT-I)

Techniques and Benefits

Cognitive Behavioral Therapy for Insomnia (CBT-I) is a structured, evidence-based approach to treating insomnia that focuses on changing the thoughts and behaviors that contribute to sleep problems. Unlike medications, CBT-I addresses the root causes of insomnia and aims to improve sleep patterns and overall sleep quality through various techniques.

Techniques:

1. **Cognitive Restructuring:** This technique involves identifying and challenging negative or unrealistic thoughts about sleep. For

example, a person who believes that not getting eight hours of sleep will ruin their day can work on altering this thought to reduce anxiety and improve sleep.

2. **Sleep Restriction Therapy:** This approach limits the time spent in bed to the actual amount of sleep obtained, thereby increasing sleep efficiency. The idea is to consolidate sleep by reducing time spent awake in bed, which can help reset the sleep-wake cycle.

3. **Stimulus Control Therapy:** This technique aims to strengthen the association between the bed and sleep. It involves guidelines such as going to bed only when sleepy, getting out of bed if unable to sleep

within 20 minutes, and using the bed only for sleep and intimacy.

4. **Relaxation Training:** Techniques such as progressive muscle relaxation, deep breathing exercises, and mindfulness meditation are used to reduce physiological arousal and promote relaxation before bedtime.

5. **Sleep Hygiene Education:** This involves educating individuals about practices that support healthy sleep, such as maintaining a consistent sleep schedule, creating a comfortable sleep environment, and avoiding stimulants like caffeine and electronic devices close to bedtime.

Benefits:

- **Long-Term Effectiveness:** CBT-I has been shown to be effective in improving sleep quality and reducing insomnia symptoms over the long term, often with lasting results even after therapy ends.

- **Non-Pharmacological:** As a non-medication-based treatment, CBT-I avoids the potential side effects and dependencies associated with sleep medications.

- **Comprehensive Approach:** By addressing the cognitive and behavioral factors contributing to insomnia, CBT-I helps individuals develop healthier sleep habits and coping strategies.

Practical Exercises

1. Sleep Diary:

Keeping a sleep diary is a fundamental exercise in CBT-I. It involves recording daily sleep patterns, including bedtime, wake time, sleep onset, and any nighttime awakenings. Tracking additional factors such as diet, caffeine intake, and daily activities can provide insights into patterns and triggers for insomnia.

How to Use:

- Record sleep and wake times daily.
- Note any factors that may impact sleep, such as stress, caffeine, or medication.

- Review the diary with a therapist to identify patterns and make adjustments to sleep habits.

2. Relaxation Techniques:

Practicing relaxation techniques helps reduce physiological arousal and prepares the body for sleep. Progressive muscle relaxation and deep breathing exercises are effective methods.

Progressive Muscle Relaxation:

- Sit or lie down in a comfortable position.
- Tense and then slowly relax each muscle group, starting from the toes and working up to the head.
- Focus on the contrast between tension and relaxation in each muscle group.

Deep Breathing Exercise:

- Sit comfortably with your back straight.

- Inhale deeply through your nose for a count of four, allowing your abdomen to rise.

- Exhale slowly through your mouth for a count of six.

- Repeat for several minutes, focusing on the rhythm of your breath.

3. Sleep Restriction Exercise:

Sleep restriction involves limiting the time spent in bed to the actual amount of sleep obtained, gradually increasing time in bed as sleep efficiency improves.

How to Implement:

- Determine your average amount of sleep per night from your sleep diary.

- Set your bedtime and wake time to match this average sleep duration.

- Gradually extend your time in bed as sleep efficiency improves, aiming for 85-90% sleep efficiency.

4. Stimulus Control Exercise:

This exercise focuses on strengthening the bed-sleep association and reducing time spent awake in bed.

How to Practice:

- Go to bed only when you feel sleepy.

- If unable to sleep within 20 minutes, get out of bed and engage in a quiet, non-stimulating activity until you feel sleepy again.

- Use the bed only for sleep and intimacy, avoiding activities like watching TV or working in bed.

5. Cognitive Restructuring Exercise:

Identify and challenge negative or unrealistic thoughts about sleep to reduce anxiety and improve sleep quality.

How to Practice:

- Record any negative thoughts related to sleep in a journal.

- Challenge these thoughts by examining evidence for and against them.

- Replace negative thoughts with more realistic and positive ones, such as "Even if I don't sleep perfectly tonight, I can still manage my day."

Cognitive Behavioral Therapy for Insomnia (CBT-I) employs various techniques and practical exercises to address and alleviate insomnia. By focusing on cognitive restructuring, behavioral changes, and relaxation strategies, CBT-I helps individuals develop healthier sleep patterns and achieve lasting improvements in sleep quality.

Chapter 7. Relaxation Techniques

Meditation and Mindfulness

Meditation and **mindfulness** are powerful relaxation techniques that can help manage stress and improve sleep quality by calming the mind and promoting relaxation.

Meditation

Meditation involves focusing the mind and eliminating distractions to achieve a state of mental clarity and calm. Regular practice can help reduce stress, anxiety, and insomnia by fostering a relaxed state conducive to sleep.

Techniques:

1. **Guided Meditation:**

- Use a guided meditation app or recording that leads you through a series of calming instructions and visualizations.

- Sit or lie down comfortably and follow the guide's instructions, focusing on relaxation and letting go of tension.

2. **Loving-Kindness Meditation:**

   - Begin by sitting quietly and focusing on your breath.

   - Silently repeat phrases such as "May I be happy, may I be healthy," and then extend these wishes to others, including loved ones and even those you have conflicts with.

o   This practice helps cultivate compassion and reduce stress.

3. **Body Scan Meditation:**

   o   Lie down or sit comfortably and close your eyes.

   o   Gradually shift your focus through different parts of your body, starting from the toes and moving upward.

   o   Notice any areas of tension or discomfort and consciously release them.

Benefits:

- Reduces stress and anxiety, which can contribute to improved sleep.

- Enhances relaxation and prepares the mind and body for sleep.
- Promotes greater awareness and presence, helping to manage racing thoughts that can interfere with falling asleep.

Mindfulness

Mindfulness involves maintaining a moment-by-moment awareness of thoughts, feelings, bodily sensations, and the surrounding environment. It encourages staying present and fully engaging with the current moment, which can help reduce stress and improve sleep.

Techniques:

1. **Mindful Breathing:**

- o Sit or lie down comfortably and focus on your breath.

- o Observe the sensation of the breath entering and leaving your body without trying to change it.

- o If your mind wanders, gently bring your focus back to your breath.

2. **Mindful Eating:**

- o Practice eating slowly and with full attention to the taste, texture, and aroma of your food.

- o This technique helps cultivate mindfulness and can reduce stress by encouraging present-moment awareness.

3. **Mindfulness Meditation:**

    - Sit comfortably with your back straight and eyes closed.

    - Focus on your breath or a mantra, observing any thoughts or sensations that arise without judgment.

    - Return your attention to your breath or mantra whenever you notice your mind wandering.

Benefits:

- Reduces stress and promotes relaxation, which can improve sleep quality.

- Helps break the cycle of negative thinking and rumination that can interfere with sleep.

- Enhances overall well-being by increasing awareness and presence.

Progressive Muscle Relaxation (PMR)

Progressive Muscle Relaxation (PMR) is a relaxation technique designed to reduce physical tension and promote deep relaxation by systematically tensing and then relaxing different muscle groups.

Techniques:

1. **Basic PMR Steps:**
   - Find a quiet, comfortable place where you can sit or lie down.
   - Begin by tensing the muscles in your toes for about 5-10 seconds, then release the tension and relax for 20-30 seconds.

- Move on to the next muscle group, such as the calves, thighs, abdomen, and so on, working your way up through the body.

- Focus on the contrast between tension and relaxation in each muscle group.

2. **Guided PMR:**

- Use a guided PMR recording or app that provides instructions for tensing and relaxing each muscle group.

- Follow the guide's prompts to practice PMR systematically and thoroughly.

Benefits:

- Reduces physical tension and promotes a state of relaxation that can improve sleep quality.

- Helps alleviate symptoms of stress and anxiety by focusing on physical relaxation.

- Can be practiced before bedtime to prepare the body and mind for sleep.

Relaxation techniques such as meditation, mindfulness, and progressive muscle relaxation offer effective ways to reduce stress and improve sleep quality. By incorporating these practices into your routine, you can enhance relaxation, manage stress, and support better sleep.

Chapter 8. Diet and Nutrition for Better Sleep

Foods to Avoid

Certain foods and beverages can negatively impact sleep quality, making it harder to fall asleep or stay asleep throughout the night. Being mindful of these can help improve overall sleep health.

1. Caffeine:

- **Sources:** Coffee, tea, energy drinks, and chocolate.

- **Impact:** Caffeine is a stimulant that can increase alertness and delay sleep onset. It can stay in the system for several hours, so it's best to avoid caffeine in the late afternoon and evening.

2. Alcohol:

- **Sources:** Beer, wine, spirits, and liquors.

- **Impact:** Although alcohol can initially make you feel drowsy, it can disrupt sleep patterns and reduce the amount of REM sleep. It can also lead to frequent awakenings during the night.

3. Heavy or Spicy Meals:

- **Sources:** Large portions of meat, rich sauces, and foods with heavy spices.

- **Impact:** Eating large or spicy meals close to bedtime can cause indigestion and discomfort, making it harder to fall asleep. It can also lead to heartburn and disrupt sleep.

4. Sugary Foods:

- **Sources:** Candy, pastries, sugary drinks, and desserts.

- **Impact:** High sugar intake can cause fluctuations in blood sugar levels, leading to disruptions in sleep. It may also contribute to insomnia by causing restless nights.

5. High-Fat Foods:

- **Sources:** Fried foods, fatty cuts of meat, and certain snacks.

- **Impact:** Foods high in fat can be harder to digest and may cause discomfort or indigestion, disrupting sleep.

Sleep-Promoting Nutrients

Certain nutrients and foods can support better sleep by promoting relaxation and regulating sleep patterns.

1. Magnesium:

- **Sources:** Nuts (especially almonds), seeds, leafy green vegetables (such as spinach), and whole grains.
- **Impact:** Magnesium plays a role in regulating the sleep-wake cycle and can help with relaxation and muscle relaxation.

2. Tryptophan:

- **Sources:** Turkey, chicken, dairy products, nuts, and seeds.

- **Impact:** Tryptophan is an amino acid that helps the body produce serotonin and melatonin, which are crucial for regulating sleep.

3. Melatonin:

- **Sources:** Cherries, grapes, and tomatoes.
- **Impact:** Melatonin is a hormone that regulates sleep-wake cycles. Consuming foods that naturally contain melatonin can support better sleep patterns.

4. Omega-3 Fatty Acids:

- **Sources:** Fatty fish (like salmon and mackerel), flaxseeds, chia seeds, and walnuts.
- **Impact:** Omega-3 fatty acids are associated with improved sleep quality and regulation.

They help reduce inflammation and support brain health, which can enhance sleep.

5. Vitamin D:

- **Sources:** Fatty fish, fortified dairy products, and exposure to sunlight.
- **Impact:** Vitamin D plays a role in regulating the sleep-wake cycle. Adequate levels of vitamin D can contribute to better sleep quality and help manage sleep disorders.

6. Herbal Teas:

- **Sources:** Chamomile tea, valerian root tea, and lavender tea.
- **Impact:** Herbal teas such as chamomile and valerian root have calming effects and may

help promote relaxation and sleep. They can be a soothing bedtime ritual.

7. Complex Carbohydrates:

- **Sources:** Whole grains, oats, and sweet potatoes.
- **Impact:** Complex carbohydrates can help increase the availability of tryptophan in the brain and promote the production of serotonin and melatonin.

Incorporating Sleep-Friendly Foods:

- **Balanced Meals:** Eating balanced meals throughout the day that include a mix of proteins, healthy fats, and complex carbohydrates can help maintain stable blood sugar levels and support restful sleep.

- **Bedtime Snacks:** Light snacks that include sleep-promoting nutrients, such as a small serving of yogurt with nuts or a piece of turkey, can be beneficial before bedtime.

- **Hydration:** Staying hydrated can support better sleep and overall well-being.

Chapter 9. Exercise and Physical Activity

Best Practices for Evening Workouts

Exercise can greatly enhance sleep quality, but the timing and type of exercise can affect how well you sleep. Here are some best practices for incorporating evening workouts:

1. Timing of Exercise:

- **Finish Early:** Aim to complete vigorous workouts at least 2-3 hours before bedtime. Intense exercise raises adrenaline levels and core body temperature, which can interfere with your ability to fall asleep.

- **Gentle Activities:** Consider engaging in gentle exercises, such as walking or stretching, closer to bedtime. These activities can help relax the body and prepare it for sleep.

2. Type of Exercise:

- **Avoid High-Intensity Workouts:** High-intensity interval training (HIIT) or heavy strength training can be stimulating and may hinder sleep if done too close to bedtime.

- **Incorporate Relaxing Exercises:** Activities like light jogging, moderate cycling, or yoga can help relax the body and mind. These exercises are less likely to interfere with sleep and can be beneficial if done in the evening.

3. Listen to Your Body:

- **Monitor Your Sleep:** Pay attention to how your evening workouts affect your sleep. If you find that exercising later in the day disrupts your sleep, consider adjusting the timing or intensity of your workouts.

- **Adapt as Needed:** Some people may find that evening exercise does not affect their sleep negatively. If this is the case for you, you may continue with your routine but remain mindful of any changes in sleep patterns.

Yoga and Stretching Routines

Yoga and stretching can be excellent for improving sleep quality by promoting relaxation and reducing muscle tension. Here are some effective yoga poses and stretching routines to incorporate into your evening routine:

1. Yoga Poses for Relaxation:

- **Child's Pose (Balasana):**
    - Kneel on the floor with your big toes touching and knees apart.
    - Sit back on your heels and extend your arms forward on the floor.
    - Rest your forehead on the mat and take deep, calming breaths.
- **Legs-Up-the-Wall Pose (Viparita Karani):**

- Lie on your back with your legs
    extended up against a wall and your
    arms at your sides.
  - Allow your lower back to relax and
    your legs to drain away tension.
  - Hold the pose for 5-10 minutes while
    focusing on your breath.
- **Reclining Bound Angle Pose (Supta Baddha Konasana):**
  - Lie on your back with your feet
    together and knees bent outward.
  - Place your hands on your abdomen or
    by your sides.
  - Use props like pillows or blankets to
    support your legs if needed.
- **Corpse Pose (Savasana):**

- Lie flat on your back with your arms and legs extended comfortably.

- Focus on your breath and let your body completely relax.

- Stay in this position for 5-10 minutes, allowing your body and mind to settle.

2. Stretching Routines for Better Sleep:

- **Neck and Shoulder Stretch:**

  - Sit or stand with your back straight. Gently tilt your head toward one shoulder and hold for 15-30 seconds.

  - Repeat on the other side.

  - Follow by gently rolling your shoulders backward and forward.

- **Forward Bend Stretch:**

  - Stand with your feet hip-width apart and slowly bend forward from your hips.

  - Let your arms hang down or grasp your elbows for a deeper stretch.

  - Hold the position for 15-30 seconds while breathing deeply.

- **Cat-Cow Stretch:**

  - Start on all fours with your wrists aligned under your shoulders and knees under your hips.

  - Inhale as you arch your back (cow pose) and exhale as you round your spine (cat pose).

- Repeat for 1-2 minutes to release tension in the back and neck.

- **Seated Forward Bend:**

    - Sit with your legs extended straight in front of you.

    - Gently reach forward toward your toes, keeping your back straight.

    - Hold for 15-30 seconds, focusing on deep, steady breathing.

Incorporating these yoga poses and stretching routines into your evening routine can help reduce stress and physical tension, promote relaxation, and improve sleep quality. Regular physical activity, combined with mindful practices, can significantly enhance your overall well-being and support better sleep.

Chapter 10. Creating the Ideal Sleep Environment

Optimizing Bedroom Conditions

Creating a sleep-friendly environment is crucial for enhancing sleep quality and ensuring restful nights. Here are key strategies for optimizing your bedroom conditions:

1. **Temperature Control:**

- **Ideal Temperature:** Keep your bedroom cool, ideally between 60-67°F (15-19°C). Cooler temperatures help lower your body's core temperature, which is conducive to sleep.

- **Adjustable Bedding:** Use breathable bedding materials like cotton or linen that help regulate temperature. Consider using a fan or an air conditioner to maintain a comfortable temperature.

2. . **Lighting:**

- **Dim Lighting:** Use dim lighting in the evening to signal to your body that it's time to wind down. Avoid bright lights or screens that emit blue light, as they can interfere with melatonin production and disrupt your sleep-wake cycle.

- **Blackout Curtains:** Install blackout curtains or shades to block out external light sources, especially if you live in a brightly lit area or have an irregular sleep schedule.

3. **Noise Control:**

- **Reduce Noise:** Minimize disruptive noises by using earplugs or a white noise machine to create a consistent, soothing sound environment. White noise can help mask sudden noises and promote deeper sleep.

- **Quiet Environment:** Ensure that your bedroom is as quiet as possible. Address any sources of noise, such as appliances or traffic, that may interfere with sleep.

4. Air Quality:

- **Ventilation:** Ensure proper airflow by keeping windows open or using an air purifier to reduce dust and allergens. Fresh air can improve sleep quality and overall comfort.

- **Humidity Control:** Maintain a moderate humidity level in your bedroom. Use a dehumidifier or humidifier if necessary to prevent discomfort caused by dry or humid air.

5. Clutter-Free Space:

- **Declutter:** Keep your bedroom clean and organized to create a calming and stress-free environment. A tidy space can help reduce anxiety and promote relaxation.
- **Designated Sleep Area:** Ensure that your bed is the primary focus of the room and avoid using it for activities other than sleep and intimacy.

The Role of Bedding and Sleep Accessories

Selecting the right bedding and sleep accessories can significantly impact your comfort and sleep quality. Here are some considerations:

1. **Mattress:**

- **Support and Comfort:** Choose a mattress that provides adequate support and comfort for your sleep style. Whether you prefer a firm, medium, or soft mattress, it should align with your body's natural curves and alleviate pressure points.

- **Quality:** Invest in a high-quality mattress that suits your needs and preferences. A good mattress can enhance sleep quality and reduce discomfort.

2. **Pillows:**

- **Supportive Pillows:** Use pillows that support your head and neck properly. The type of pillow (e.g., memory foam, down, or ergonomic) should align with your sleeping position (back, side, or stomach).

- **Regular Replacement:** Replace pillows every 1-2 years or when they lose their shape and support.

3. **Bedding:**

- **Breathable Materials:** Opt for bedding made from natural, breathable materials like cotton or bamboo that wick away moisture and regulate temperature.

- **Comfort and Cleanliness:** Ensure that your bedding is comfortable and clean. Regularly wash sheets and pillowcases to maintain a fresh and hygienic sleep environment.

4. **Sleep Accessories:**

- **Eye Masks:** Use an eye mask to block out light and help signal to your body that it's time to sleep, especially if you are sensitive to light.

- **Sleep Aids:** Consider using aromatherapy with essential oils like lavender, which can promote relaxation and improve sleep quality.

- **Weighted Blankets:** For some individuals, weighted blankets can provide a sense of security and reduce anxiety, leading to improved sleep.

5. Bed Placement:

- **Optimal Position:** Position your bed to create a harmonious flow in the room. Avoid placing it directly in line with the door or under a window to minimize disturbances and enhance feelings of safety and comfort.

Chapter 11. The Impact of Technology on Sleep

Managing Screen Time

Technology plays a significant role in modern life, but excessive screen time, especially before bed, can adversely affect sleep quality. Managing screen time effectively can help improve sleep.

1. Establish a Digital Curfew:

- **Screen-Free Time:** Set a specific time in the evening, ideally 1-2 hours before bedtime, to disconnect from all screens, including smartphones, tablets, and computers.

- **Bedtime Routine:** Use the time before bed for relaxing activities that do not involve screens, such as reading a book, taking a warm bath, or practicing relaxation techniques.

2. Create a Sleep-Friendly Environment:

- **Designate Tech-Free Zones:** Keep electronic devices out of the bedroom to create a more restful environment. Use your bedroom solely for sleep and relaxation to strengthen the mental association between your bed and rest.

- **Limit Notifications:** Turn off non-essential notifications on your devices to minimize disruptions and reduce the urge to check your phone before bed.

3. Use Technology Wisely:

- **Night Mode:** Many devices offer a "night mode" or "dark mode" that reduces screen brightness and changes the color temperature to warmer tones. Use these features in the evening to lessen the impact on sleep.

- **Screen Time Apps:** Utilize apps or built-in features that track and limit screen time. These tools can help you monitor usage and set limits to prevent excessive screen time.

Blue Light:

1. Understanding Blue Light:

- **Definition:** Blue light is a type of high-energy visible (HEV) light emitted by screens, including smartphones, tablets, computers, and LED lighting.

- **Impact on Sleep:** Blue light exposure, especially in the evening, can interfere with the production of melatonin, the hormone responsible for regulating sleep. This disruption can delay sleep onset and reduce sleep quality.

2. **Effects of Blue Light:**

- **Disruption of Circadian Rhythm:** Blue light exposure in the evening can shift your circadian rhythm, making it harder to fall asleep at the desired time and potentially leading to sleep disorders.

- **Reduced Sleep Quality:** Prolonged exposure to blue light before bedtime can lead to lighter sleep and increased nighttime awakenings, impacting overall sleep quality.

3. **Mitigating Blue Light Exposure:**

- **Use Blue Light Filters:** Many devices come with built-in blue light filters or "night mode" settings that reduce the amount of

blue light emitted. Enable these features
during evening hours.

- **Wear Blue Light Glasses:** Specialized blue
  light blocking glasses can help reduce blue
  light exposure from screens. Consider using
  them if you must use devices before bedtime.

- **Adjust Lighting:** Use dim, warm-colored
  lighting in the evening to minimize blue light
  exposure from home lighting. Opt for lamps
  with yellow or red light bulbs rather than
  bright, cool-toned LED lights.

4. **Alternative Solutions:**

- **Physical Books:** Opt for reading physical
  books or using an e-reader with a non-backlit

screen in the evening to avoid blue light
exposure.

- **Relaxation Techniques:** Incorporate
  non-screen-based relaxation activities into
  your pre-sleep routine, such as meditation,
  journaling, or listening to calming music.

Managing screen time and understanding the
impact of blue light are essential for improving
sleep quality. By establishing a digital curfew,
utilizing blue light filters, and incorporating
alternative pre-sleep activities, you can mitigate the
negative effects of technology and support better
sleep health.

Chapter 12. Natural Remedies and Supplements

Herbal Teas and Essential Oils

Herbal Teas:

Herbal teas can be a soothing way to promote relaxation and improve sleep quality. Many herbal teas contain compounds that can help calm the mind and prepare the body for restful sleep.

1. Chamomile Tea:

- **Benefits:** Chamomile is known for its calming properties and is often used to reduce anxiety and promote relaxation. It contains apigenin, an antioxidant that may help induce sleep.

- **How to Use:** Drink a cup of chamomile tea about 30 minutes before bedtime. Choose high-quality, caffeine-free chamomile tea for the best results.

2. **Lavender Tea:**

- **Benefits:** Lavender has been shown to have soothing effects and can help alleviate symptoms of anxiety and insomnia. It may improve sleep quality and reduce the time it takes to fall asleep.

- **How to Use:** Brew lavender tea from dried lavender flowers or use a pre-packaged lavender tea blend. Consume about an hour before bed.

3. **Valerian Root Tea:**

- **Benefits:** Valerian root is known for its sedative properties and has been used historically to treat insomnia and anxiety. It may help improve sleep latency and overall sleep quality.

- **How to Use:** Drink valerian root tea approximately 30-60 minutes before bedtime. Be aware that valerian may have a strong taste.

Essential Oils:

Essential oils can be used aromatically or topically to promote relaxation and support better sleep.

1. **Lavender Oil:**

- **Benefits:** Lavender essential oil is commonly used to reduce stress and promote restful sleep. Its calming aroma can help lower anxiety levels and improve sleep quality.

- **How to Use:** Diffuse lavender oil in your bedroom, add a few drops to a pillow, or apply diluted lavender oil to your wrists or neck before bedtime.

2. **Roman Chamomile Oil:**

- **Benefits:** Roman chamomile essential oil has soothing properties that can help alleviate stress and promote relaxation. It is often used to support better sleep and calm an overactive mind.

- **How to Use:** Diffuse Roman chamomile oil or add a few drops to a carrier oil and apply it to your skin.

3. Cedarwood Oil:

- **Benefits:** Cedarwood essential oil has calming and grounding effects that can help promote relaxation and improve sleep quality. It is also thought to have sedative properties.

- **How to Use:** Diffuse cedarwood oil in the evening or mix it with a carrier oil and apply it to your feet or neck.

Melatonin and Other Supplements

Melatonin:

Melatonin is a hormone that helps regulate the sleep-wake cycle. It is commonly used as a supplement to improve sleep quality and address issues like insomnia or jet lag.

1. **Benefits:**

- **Sleep Regulation:** Melatonin helps signal to the body that it's time to sleep, making it useful for managing sleep disorders and adjusting to time zone changes.

- **Sleep Quality:** Supplementing with melatonin may help improve sleep onset, duration, and overall quality, especially in individuals with low melatonin levels.

2. **How to Use:**

- **Dosage:** Melatonin supplements are typically available in doses ranging from 0.5 to 5 mg. Start with a low dose and adjust as needed based on effectiveness and tolerance.

- **Timing:** Take melatonin approximately 30-60 minutes before bedtime. It is best used in conjunction with good sleep hygiene practices.

Other Supplements:

1. **Magnesium:**

- **Benefits:** Magnesium supports relaxation by regulating neurotransmitters and muscle function. It can help alleviate symptoms of insomnia and improve sleep quality.

- **How to Use:** Consider taking magnesium supplements in the evening, preferably in a form that is easily absorbed, such as magnesium citrate or glycinate.

2. Valerian Root:

- **Benefits:** Valerian root is known for its sedative effects and can help improve sleep latency and quality. It may be particularly helpful for those with anxiety-related sleep disturbances.

- **How to Use:** Valerian root is available in capsule, tincture, or tea form. Follow the dosage instructions on the product label.

3. Glycine:

- **Benefits:** Glycine is an amino acid that has been shown to improve sleep quality and reduce the time it takes to fall asleep. It may also help regulate body temperature during sleep.

- **How to Use:** Glycine supplements can be taken before bedtime. The typical dosage ranges from 1 to 3 grams.

4. L-Theanine:

- **Benefits:** L-Theanine is an amino acid found in tea leaves that promotes relaxation and reduces stress without causing drowsiness. It can help improve sleep quality by reducing anxiety and promoting

calmness.

- **How to Use:** L-Theanine supplements are

  usually taken in doses of 100-200 mg before

  bedtime.

Natural remedies and supplements, including herbal teas, essential oils, melatonin, and other supplements, can support better sleep by promoting relaxation and addressing sleep disruptions. Incorporate these remedies thoughtfully, considering individual needs and preferences, to enhance overall sleep quality.

Chapter 13. Sleep Hygiene Practices

Establishing a Bedtime Routine

A consistent bedtime routine can signal to your body that it's time to wind down and prepare for sleep. Here's how to establish an effective bedtime routine:

1. **Create a Relaxing Pre-Sleep Ritual:**

- **Wind-Down Activities:** Engage in calming activities before bed to help transition from the day's stress to a state of relaxation. Consider reading a book, taking a warm bath, practicing gentle yoga, or listening to soothing music.

- **Avoid Stimulating Activities:** Steer clear of stimulating activities such as watching intense TV shows, engaging in vigorous exercise, or working on tasks that may increase stress or alertness.

2. Follow a Consistent Routine:

- **Bedtime Ritual:** Develop a series of calming actions that signal to your body that it's time to sleep. This could include brushing your teeth, dimming the lights, and performing relaxation exercises.

- **Predictable Timing:** Go to bed and wake up at the same time every day, even on weekends. This consistency reinforces your body's internal clock and improves overall sleep quality.

3. Create a Sleep-Inducing Environment:

- **Comfortable Setting:** Ensure your bedroom is conducive to sleep by making it cool, dark, and quiet. Invest in comfortable bedding and a supportive mattress.

- **Limit Distractions:** Keep electronic devices out of the bedroom and create a space dedicated solely to sleep. This helps reinforce the association between your bed and rest.

4. Incorporate Relaxation Techniques:

- **Mindfulness and Breathing Exercises:** Include mindfulness practices or deep breathing exercises in your bedtime routine to calm the mind and reduce pre-sleep anxiety.

- **Progressive Muscle Relaxation:** Practice progressive muscle relaxation to ease physical tension and prepare your body for rest.

Tips for a Consistent Sleep Schedule

Maintaining a consistent sleep schedule is key to regulating your body's internal clock and improving sleep quality. Here are some tips for achieving consistency:

1. Set a Fixed Sleep and Wake Time:

- **Regular Timing:** Choose a specific time to go to bed and wake up each day, and stick to this schedule as closely as possible. Consistency reinforces your body's circadian rhythm and helps regulate sleep patterns.

- **Adjust Gradually:** If you need to shift your sleep schedule, make gradual adjustments by 15-30 minutes at a time. Sudden changes can disrupt your internal clock and affect sleep quality.

2. Use Sleep Aids Wisely:

- **Alarms:** Set a gentle alarm to wake up at the same time each morning. Avoid using snooze buttons, as they can disrupt your sleep cycle and make it harder to wake up feeling refreshed.

- **Light Exposure:** Expose yourself to natural light in the morning to help regulate your circadian rhythm. Spend time outside or open your curtains to let in sunlight.

3. **Limit Naps:**

- **Nap Duration:** If you need to nap during the day, keep it brief (20-30 minutes) and avoid napping late in the afternoon or evening. Long or late naps can interfere with nighttime sleep and disrupt your sleep schedule.

4. **Be Mindful of Evening Activities:**

- **Avoid Stimulants:** Reduce caffeine and alcohol intake in the hours leading up to bedtime, as these substances can interfere with sleep quality and make it harder to adhere to a consistent schedule.

- **Evening Routine:** Develop a calming evening routine to signal to your body that it's time to wind down. Engage in relaxing activities and avoid stimulating screens and bright lights.

5. **Manage Stress and Anxiety:**

- **Relaxation Techniques:** Practice relaxation techniques such as meditation, deep breathing, or journaling to manage stress and anxiety that may impact your ability to maintain a consistent sleep schedule.

- **Problem-Solving:** Address any concerns or worries before bedtime to prevent them from interfering with your ability to fall asleep and stay asleep.

6. **Stay Active:**

- **Regular Exercise:** Incorporate regular physical activity into your routine, but avoid vigorous exercise close to bedtime. Exercise can help regulate your sleep patterns and improve overall sleep quality.

Establishing a bedtime routine and maintaining a consistent sleep schedule are essential for improving sleep hygiene and overall sleep quality. By creating a relaxing pre-sleep environment, setting fixed sleep and wake times, and managing evening activities, you can support better sleep and overall well-being.

Chapter 14. The Role of Mental Health

Addressing Depression and Anxiety

Mental health conditions such as depression and anxiety can significantly impact sleep quality and contribute to insomnia. Addressing these conditions is crucial for improving overall sleep and well-being.

1. Understanding the Connection:

- **Impact on Sleep:** Depression and anxiety can lead to difficulties falling asleep, staying asleep, or experiencing restful sleep. Symptoms such as racing thoughts, excessive worry, and low mood can disrupt sleep patterns and exacerbate sleep disorders.

- **Sleep Disruptions:** Poor sleep can, in turn, worsen symptoms of depression and anxiety, creating a cycle of sleep problems and mental health issues.

2. Strategies for Managing Depression and Anxiety:

- **Cognitive Behavioral Therapy (CBT):** CBT is an evidence-based therapy that can help manage both depression and anxiety. It focuses on identifying and changing negative thought patterns and behaviors that contribute to mental health issues and sleep disturbances.

- **Mindfulness and Relaxation:** Practices such as mindfulness meditation, deep breathing exercises, and progressive muscle relaxation can help reduce stress and anxiety, promoting a sense of calm and improving sleep.

- **Healthy Lifestyle Choices:** Incorporate regular physical activity, balanced nutrition, and adequate hydration into your daily routine to support mental health and improve sleep quality.

- **Sleep Hygiene:** Follow good sleep hygiene practices, such as establishing a consistent sleep routine and creating a relaxing bedtime environment, to support better sleep and overall mental health.

3. **Self-Care and Support:**

- **Develop Coping Skills:** Learn and practice coping strategies to manage stress and anxiety. Techniques such as journaling, engaging in hobbies, and connecting with supportive friends or family can help alleviate symptoms.

- **Set Realistic Goals:** Set achievable goals for managing mental health and sleep. Gradual improvements in daily habits and routines can lead to positive changes in both areas.

Seeking Professional Help

When self-care strategies and lifestyle changes are not sufficient, seeking professional help is important for effectively managing depression, anxiety, and related sleep issues.

1. **Types of Professional Help:**

- **Mental Health Professionals:** Consider consulting a licensed mental health professional, such as a psychologist, psychiatrist, or clinical social worker, for an accurate diagnosis and personalized treatment plan.

- **Therapists and Counselors:** Therapists and counselors can provide individual or group therapy sessions to address underlying mental health issues and offer support in managing symptoms.

- **Medical Doctors:** For individuals with more severe symptoms or complex cases, a primary care physician or psychiatrist may provide medication management and coordinate care with other specialists.

**2. Treatment Options:

- **Medication:** Medications such as antidepressants or anti-anxiety medications may be prescribed by a healthcare provider to manage symptoms of depression or anxiety. Medication should be used under the guidance of a healthcare professional.

- **Therapeutic Interventions:** Therapies such as CBT, dialectical behavior therapy (DBT), or acceptance and commitment therapy (ACT) can help address cognitive and emotional aspects of mental health conditions and improve sleep.

- **Behavioral Strategies:** Professional guidance on behavioral strategies, such as sleep restriction therapy or stimulus control therapy, can be beneficial in managing insomnia and improving sleep patterns.

3. Support Systems:

- **Support Groups:** Joining support groups or community resources can provide a sense of connection and shared experience. Peer support can be valuable in managing mental health challenges and improving overall well-being.

- **Family and Friends:** Engaging with supportive family members and friends can offer emotional support and encouragement throughout the process of managing mental health and sleep issues.

4. Monitoring Progress:

- **Regular Check-Ins:** Schedule regular follow-up appointments with healthcare providers to monitor progress, adjust treatment plans as needed, and address any concerns.

- **Track Symptoms:** Keep track of symptoms and sleep patterns to provide accurate information to healthcare providers and evaluate the effectiveness of treatment strategies.

Addressing mental health conditions such as depression and anxiety is essential for improving sleep quality and overall well-being. By utilizing self-care strategies, seeking professional help, and engaging with support systems, individuals can effectively manage mental health challenges and enhance their sleep and quality of life.

Chapter 15. Medical Treatments and Medications

Prescription Sleep Aids

Prescription sleep aids can be helpful for managing severe or persistent insomnia, especially when other treatments have not been effective. Here's an overview of common prescription sleep aids:

1. Benzodiazepines:

- **Examples:** Temazepam (Restoril), Lorazepam (Ativan), Diazepam (Valium).
- **Benefits:** These medications can help induce sleep and reduce anxiety. They work by enhancing the effects of a neurotransmitter called gamma-aminobutyric acid (GABA), which has calming effects on the brain.

- **Considerations:** Benzodiazepines are typically used for short-term management due to the risk of dependence, tolerance, and withdrawal symptoms. They can also cause next-day drowsiness and impair cognitive function.

2. Non-Benzodiazepine Hypnotics:

- **Examples:** Zolpidem (Ambien), Eszopiclone (Lunesta), Zaleplon (Sonata).
- **Benefits:** These medications are designed to improve sleep initiation and maintenance. They generally have a shorter duration of action compared to benzodiazepines, which can reduce the risk of morning drowsiness.

- **Considerations:** Non-benzodiazepine hypnotics can still lead to dependence or tolerance if used long-term. Potential side effects include dizziness, headache, and sleepwalking.

3. Melatonin Receptor Agonists:

- **Examples:** Ramelteon (Rozerem), Tasimelteon (Hetlioz).

- **Benefits:** These drugs mimic the action of melatonin, a natural sleep hormone, and are used to regulate the sleep-wake cycle. They are particularly useful for conditions like delayed sleep phase disorder.

- **Considerations:** Melatonin receptor agonists are generally considered safe and have fewer side effects compared to other sleep aids. However, they may not be as effective for all types of insomnia.

4. Antidepressants

- **Examples:** Trazodone (Desyrel), Doxepin (Silenor).
- **Mechanism:** These medications, primarily used for depression, have sedative effects that can help with insomnia.
- **Efficacy:** Often used when insomnia is associated with depression or anxiety.
- **Side Effects:** May include drowsiness, dry mouth, and potential weight gain.

B. Over-the-Counter Medications

1. Antihistamines

- **Examples:** Diphenhydramine (Benadryl), Doxylamine (Unisom).

- **Mechanism:** These drugs block histamine receptors in the brain, which can promote drowsiness.

- **Efficacy:** Useful for occasional insomnia, but not recommended for long-term use.

- **Side Effects:** May cause dry mouth, constipation, and next-day drowsiness.

2. Melatonin Supplements

- **Examples:** Available in various doses over-the-counter.

- **Mechanism:** Provides supplemental melatonin to help regulate the sleep-wake cycle.

- **Efficacy:** Can be helpful for certain types of insomnia, particularly those related to circadian rhythm disorders.

- **Side Effects:** Generally minimal, but can include dizziness or nausea.

Considerations and Guidelines

1. Safety and Side Effects

When considering pharmacological treatments for insomnia, it's essential to weigh the benefits against potential side effects. For chronic use, medications with a lower risk of dependency and adverse effects are preferred. Regular follow-ups and evaluations are crucial to monitor efficacy and manage side effects.

2. Individualized Treatment

Treatment should be tailored to the individual, taking into account the underlying cause of insomnia, patient preferences, and any coexisting medical conditions. For instance, patients with a history of substance abuse may need alternative treatments to avoid potential dependency issues.

3. Combination Therapies

In some cases, a combination of medications and behavioral therapies may provide the best outcomes. For example, CBT-I can be used alongside pharmacological treatments to enhance overall effectiveness.

Medical treatments and medications for insomnia offer a range of options to help individuals achieve better sleep. While medications can provide symptomatic relief, they should be used judiciously and typically in conjunction with non-pharmacological therapies. Ongoing research and advancements in the field continue to improve the understanding and management of insomnia, providing hope for more effective and personalized treatment strategies in the future.

Chapter 16: Tracking and Monitoring Sleep

Introduction

Effective management of sleep disorders such as insomnia requires accurate tracking and monitoring of sleep patterns.

By systematically recording sleep-related data, individuals and healthcare providers can gain valuable insights into sleep behavior, identify patterns, and tailor interventions.

This chapter explores two primary tools for tracking and monitoring sleep: sleep diaries and wearable sleep trackers.

Using Sleep Diaries

Overview

A sleep diary is a self-report tool used to record various aspects of sleep and wakefulness over time. It is a simple yet effective way to monitor sleep patterns and can help identify factors that may contribute to sleep disturbances.

Components of a Sleep Diary

1. Sleep Onset Time: Record the time when attempting to fall asleep.

 2. Wake Time: Note the time of awakening, both in the morning and during the night.

3. Number and Duration of Nighttime Awakenings: Track any instances of waking during the night and how long it takes to return to sleep.

4. Morning Wakefulness: Record how refreshed or tired one feels upon waking.

5. Daily Activities: Include information on exercise, caffeine intake, alcohol consumption, and medication use.

6. Naps: Record the duration and timing of any daytime naps.

7. Bedtime Routines: Note any pre-sleep activities, such as reading or screen time.

Benefits

1. Identifying Patterns: A sleep diary helps to identify consistent patterns and triggers related to sleep disturbances.

 2. Personalized Insights: Provides a personalized view of sleep habits that can guide adjustments in lifestyle or bedtime routines.

 3. Communication Tool: Facilitates communication between patients and healthcare providers, offering a detailed account of sleep issues for better diagnosis and treatment planning.

Limitations

1. Accuracy: Data may be affected by subjective reporting and recall biases. **2. Time-Consuming:**

Maintaining a sleep diary requires consistent effort and attention to detail.

Wearable Sleep Trackers

Overview

Wearable sleep trackers are electronic devices designed to monitor and record various sleep-related metrics. These devices can provide detailed, real-time data about sleep patterns, often incorporating advanced technology and algorithms to analyze sleep quality.

Types of Wearable Sleep Trackers

1. Fitness Trackers: Devices such as Fitbit, Garmin, and Apple Watch that offer basic sleep monitoring features. **2. Specialized Sleep**

Trackers: Dedicated devices like the Oura Ring and the WHOOP Strap, which focus specifically on sleep tracking and recovery.

Key Metrics Monitored

1. Sleep Duration: Measures the total amount of sleep obtained.

2. Sleep Stages: Tracks different stages of sleep, including light, deep, and REM sleep.

 3. Sleep Latency: Records the time taken to fall asleep.

4. Sleep Efficiency: Calculates the percentage of time spent asleep relative to time spent in bed.

5. Heart Rate Variability: Monitors changes in heart rate, which can indicate overall sleep quality and recovery.

Benefits

1. Objective Data: Provides quantitative, objective data on sleep patterns, which can complement subjective reports.

2. Real-Time Monitoring: Allows for continuous tracking and immediate feedback.

3. Long-Term Trends: Facilitates the observation of long-term sleep trends and patterns.

4. Integration: Often integrates with mobile apps to provide detailed reports and insights.

Limitations

1. Accuracy Variability: The accuracy of sleep tracking can vary between devices and may not always align with clinical sleep studies.

2. Comfort and Wearability: Some devices may be uncomfortable or intrusive, potentially affecting sleep quality.

3. Data Interpretation: Requires careful interpretation of data, as the technology may not capture all aspects of sleep disorders.

Both sleep diaries and wearable sleep trackers offer valuable tools for tracking and monitoring sleep. Sleep diaries provide subjective, detailed insights into sleep patterns and behaviors, while wearable trackers offer objective, real-time data. Combining both methods can enhance the overall understanding of sleep issues, aiding in more effective management and treatment strategies. Regular tracking and monitoring are essential for identifying sleep problems and making informed decisions about interventions and lifestyle changes.

Chapter 17: Dealing with Shift Work and Jet Lag

Introduction

Shift work and travel across time zones can significantly disrupt sleep patterns, leading to issues such as insomnia, fatigue, and reduced overall well-being. This chapter provides strategies to manage sleep disruptions associated with shift work and jet lag, focusing on practical approaches to minimize their impact and maintain healthy sleep habits.

Strategies for Night Shift Workers

- **. Optimize Sleep Environment**

1. Darkness: Use blackout curtains or an eye mask to create a dark sleeping environment during the day.

2. Quiet: Employ earplugs or white noise machines to block out daytime noise.

 3. Cool Temperature: Maintain a cool and comfortable room temperature to enhance sleep quality.

- **Establish a Consistent Sleep Schedule**

1. Regularity: Try to go to bed and wake up at the same times each day, even on days off, to regulate your body's internal clock.

2. Pre-Sleep Routine: Develop a relaxing pre-sleep routine to signal to your body that it's time to wind down. This might include activities like reading or taking a warm bath.

- **Manage Light Exposure**

1. Light Exposure During Shifts: Maximize exposure to bright light during night shifts to help adjust your body clock. Specialized light therapy lamps can be useful.

2. Light Exposure Before Sleep: Minimize exposure to bright light, especially blue light from screens, before your sleep period. Use blue light filters on devices or wear blue light blocking glasses.

- **Nutritional and Lifestyle Adjustments**

1. Meal Timing: Eat meals at consistent times and consider having a light meal before the night shift. Avoid heavy, rich foods close to bedtime.

2. Caffeine Use: Limit caffeine intake to the early part of your shift to avoid interference with sleep.

- **Exercise**

1. Physical Activity: Engage in regular exercise, but avoid vigorous activity close to your sleep time. Exercise can help regulate your sleep patterns and reduce stress.

Overcoming Travel-Related Sleep Issues

- **Pre-Trip Preparation**

1. Gradual Adjustment: If possible, gradually shift your sleep schedule to match your destination's time zone before traveling. Adjust your bedtime and wake-up time by 30 minutes to an hour each day leading up to the trip.

2. Light Exposure: Adjust your light exposure according to your new time zone. Spend time in natural light in the morning if traveling east or in the afternoon if traveling west.

- **During Travel**

1. Hydration: Stay well-hydrated and avoid excessive alcohol and caffeine, as these can disrupt sleep.

 2. Sleep Aids: Consider using sleep aids like eye masks, neck pillows, or noise-canceling headphones to improve sleep quality on long flights or train rides.

- **Post-Arrival Strategies**

1. Adapt to Local Time: Immediately adopt the local schedule for meals and sleep. Try to stay awake until the local bedtime to help adjust your internal clock.

2. Exposure to Daylight: Spend time outdoors in natural daylight upon arrival. This helps reset your circadian rhythm and adapt to the new time zone.

3. Nap Wisely: If you need to nap after arrival, limit it to 20-30 minutes and avoid napping late in the day to prevent interference with nighttime sleep.

- **Sleep Hygiene**

1. Create a Comfortable Sleep Environment: Ensure your sleep environment at your destination is conducive to rest—dark, quiet, and cool.

2. Relaxation Techniques: Practice relaxation techniques such as deep breathing, meditation, or progressive muscle relaxation to ease into sleep.

Managing sleep disruptions from shift work and jet lag requires a combination of strategic planning, environmental adjustments, and lifestyle modifications. By implementing these strategies, individuals can better cope with the challenges posed by irregular work hours and travel, ultimately leading to improved sleep quality and overall well-being. Regularly assessing and adjusting these strategies can help maintain a stable sleep pattern and reduce the impact of external disruptions.

Chapter 18: Insomnia in Children and Teens

Insomnia in children and adolescents presents unique challenges and requires tailored approaches to effectively address and manage. Sleep disturbances in this age group can impact cognitive development, emotional regulation, and overall health. This chapter explores the specific challenges associated with insomnia in children and teens and provides strategies for establishing healthy sleep habits from an early age.

Unique Challenges and Solutions

- **Developmental Factors**

1. Sleep Patterns: Children and teens undergo significant changes in sleep patterns as they grow.

Younger children often require more sleep, while teenagers may experience shifts in their sleep-wake cycles due to hormonal changes.

2. School and Extracurricular Demands: Academic pressures, extracurricular activities, and social commitments can interfere with sleep schedules and contribute to insomnia.

- **Behavioral and Psychological Factors**

1. Anxiety and Stress: Academic pressure, social issues, and family dynamics can contribute to sleep problems. Teens, in particular, may experience heightened stress related to exams, peer relationships, and identity formation.

2. Technology Use: Excessive use of screens before bedtime can disrupt sleep due to the blue light emitted by devices, which interferes with melatonin production.

- **Medical and Physical Factors**

1. Sleep Disorders: Conditions such as sleep apnea, restless legs syndrome, and narcolepsy can affect sleep quality. Proper diagnosis and management of these conditions are crucial.

2. Health Conditions: Chronic illnesses, medication side effects, and conditions like ADHD can impact sleep patterns.

Solutions and Strategies

1. Cognitive Behavioral Therapy for Insomnia (CBT-I): Adaptations of CBT-I can be effective for children and teens, focusing on modifying negative sleep-related thoughts and behaviors in a developmentally appropriate way.

2. Consistent Sleep Routine: Establishing a regular bedtime and wake-up time, even on weekends, helps regulate the internal clock. A predictable bedtime routine can signal to the body that it is time to wind down.

3. Technology Management: Limit screen time before bed and ensure devices are used in a way that does not interfere with sleep. Consider implementing a "tech-free" hour before bedtime.

4. Stress Management Techniques: Incorporate relaxation techniques such as deep breathing, mindfulness, or progressive muscle relaxation to help manage stress and anxiety that may affect sleep.

5. Sleep Environment: Create a comfortable, quiet, and dark sleep environment. Using a nightlight, if needed, and ensuring a comfortable mattress and pillows can enhance sleep quality.

Establishing Healthy Sleep Habits Early

- **Setting the Foundation**

1. Establish Consistent Routines: From an early age, establish regular sleep and wake times. Consistency helps regulate the child's internal clock and fosters good sleep habits.

2. Positive Sleep Associations: Create a positive association with sleep by developing a calming bedtime routine. Activities such as reading a book, taking a warm bath, or listening to soothing music can signal that it's time to wind down.

- **Educating About Sleep Hygiene**

1. Importance of Sleep: Educate children and teens about the importance of sleep for their health, mood, and performance. Understanding the benefits can motivate them to prioritize good sleep habits.

2. Healthy Habits: Promote habits such as limiting caffeine intake, avoiding heavy meals close to bedtime, and maintaining an appropriate balance between screen time and physical activity.

- **Role of Parents and Caregivers**

1. Modeling Behavior: Parents and caregivers should model good sleep hygiene practices. Consistent sleep routines and healthy sleep behaviors set a positive example for children and teens.

2. Support and Encouragement: Offer support and encouragement in maintaining healthy sleep habits. Address any sleep-related issues or concerns promptly and seek professional help if needed.

- **Professional Guidance**

1. Regular Check-Ups: Regular medical check-ups can help identify and address any sleep-related issues early. Discuss any concerns about sleep patterns or behaviors with a healthcare provider.

2. Referral to Specialists: If insomnia persists despite implementing healthy sleep habits, consider seeking guidance from a sleep specialist or psychologist who has experience working with children and teens.

Addressing insomnia in children and teens requires an understanding of the unique developmental, behavioral, and environmental factors that impact sleep. Regular monitoring, education, and professional support are key to effectively managing sleep issues in this age group.

Chapter 19: Success Stories and Case Studies

Introduction

Success stories and case studies offer valuable insights into how individuals overcome insomnia and related sleep disorders. By examining real-life experiences, we can understand effective strategies, common challenges, and key lessons that can be applied to similar situations. This chapter presents a range of success stories and case studies, highlighting the diverse approaches to managing insomnia and the outcomes achieved.

Real-Life Experiences

1. Case Study: Laura's Journey with Chronic Insomnia

Background: Laura, a 35-year-old marketing executive, had struggled with chronic insomnia for over five years. Her primary issues included difficulty falling asleep, frequent awakenings, and non-restorative sleep. Despite trying various over-the-counter sleep aids, Laura's sleep problems persisted, impacting her work performance and overall quality of life.

Approach: Laura decided to pursue Cognitive Behavioral Therapy for Insomnia (CBT-I) after a referral from her primary care physician. The therapy included:

- **Sleep Education:** Learning about sleep hygiene and the impact of her behaviors on sleep.

- **Cognitive Restructuring:** Addressing her anxiety about sleep and changing her negative beliefs.

- **Behavioral Techniques:** Implementing sleep restriction and stimulus control strategies.

Outcome: After eight weeks of CBT-I, Laura reported significant improvements in sleep quality. She experienced fewer awakenings, reduced sleep latency, and felt more refreshed upon waking. Her work performance and overall mood also improved. Laura's success underscores the effectiveness of CBT-I in treating chronic insomnia.

2. Case Study: Mike's Adjustment to Night Shifts

Background: Mike, a 45-year-old paramedic, worked night shifts that disrupted his sleep pattern. He struggled with fatigue and difficulty adjusting his sleep schedule between shifts. Traditional sleep aids were ineffective and caused undesirable side effects.

Approach: Mike adopted several strategies to manage his shift work-related sleep issues:

- **Sleep Environment:** Invested in blackout curtains and a white noise machine for his sleep space.
- **Light Exposure:** Used a light therapy box during night shifts and avoided bright screens before sleep.

- **Consistent Routine:** Maintained a consistent sleep schedule, even on days off, to stabilize his internal clock.

Outcome: Mike successfully adapted to his night shifts, reporting improved sleep quality and reduced fatigue. His ability to manage light exposure and create a conducive sleep environment played a critical role in his success. This case highlights the importance of tailored strategies for shift workers.

3. Case Study: Emma's Recovery from Jet Lag

Background: Emma, a 28-year-old consultant, frequently traveled across time zones for work. She experienced severe jet lag, with symptoms including insomnia, fatigue, and difficulty concentrating.

Approach: Emma implemented several strategies to mitigate jet lag:

- **Pre-Trip Adjustments:** Gradually shifted her sleep schedule to match her destination's time zone.

- **During Travel:** Stayed hydrated, used an eye mask, and avoided caffeine and alcohol during flights.

- **Post-Arrival:** Exposed herself to natural light upon arrival and adjusted to the local schedule immediately.

Outcome: Emma reported a significant reduction in jet lag symptoms and improved sleep quality. Her proactive approach to adjusting her sleep schedule and managing travel-related factors contributed to a smoother transition between time zones. This case demonstrates the effectiveness of strategic planning in overcoming travel-related sleep issues.

Lessons Learned

1. Importance of Personalized Approaches

Each individual's experience with insomnia is unique, and successful outcomes often depend on personalized treatment plans. Whether through behavioral therapies, environmental adjustments, or lifestyle changes, tailoring strategies to specific needs is crucial.

2. Role of Comprehensive Strategies

Addressing insomnia often requires a multifaceted approach. Combining different strategies, such as cognitive-behavioral therapy, environmental modifications, and lifestyle changes, can yield better results than relying on a single solution.

3. Value of Professional Guidance

In many cases, seeking professional help, such as consulting with sleep specialists or therapists, can provide targeted interventions and support. Professional guidance can be instrumental in diagnosing underlying issues and developing effective treatment plans.

4. Importance of Consistency and Patience

Managing insomnia and achieving better sleep often requires consistent effort and patience. Adhering to recommended strategies and giving them time to take effect is essential for long-term success.

5. Adaptability and Flexibility

Successful management of insomnia involves adapting strategies to changing circumstances, such as shift work or travel. Being flexible and open to adjusting approaches as needed can enhance overall effectiveness.

Success stories and case studies provide valuable insights into overcoming insomnia and improving sleep quality. These insights can guide individuals and healthcare providers in developing and implementing successful interventions for managing insomnia and related sleep disorders.

Chapter 20: Conclusion: Embracing Restful Nights

Achieving restful nights is crucial for overall well-being, as sleep affects physical health, mental clarity, and emotional stability. This concluding chapter consolidates key insights into long-term strategies and ongoing practices to maintain optimal sleep health. By embracing these approaches, individuals can foster enduring sleep improvements and enhance their quality of life.

Long-Term Strategies

- **Establishing and Maintaining a Consistent Sleep Routine**

1. Regular Sleep Schedule: Adhere to a consistent bedtime and wake-up time, even on weekends, to regulate your internal clock. Consistency helps reinforce healthy sleep patterns and improve overall sleep quality.

2. Pre-Sleep Routine: Develop a relaxing pre-sleep routine to signal your body that it's time to wind down. This routine might include activities like reading, taking a warm bath, or practicing relaxation techniques.

- **Creating a Sleep-Conducive Environment**

1. Optimize Sleep Conditions: Ensure your sleep environment is dark, quiet, and cool. Invest in a comfortable mattress and pillows, and use blackout curtains or a sleep mask to minimize light exposure.

2. Manage Noise: Use white noise machines or earplugs to block out disruptive noises and create a more peaceful sleep environment.

- **Prioritizing Sleep Hygiene**

1. Healthy Lifestyle Choices: Maintain a balanced diet, exercise regularly, and avoid excessive caffeine, nicotine, and alcohol, especially close to bedtime.

2. Screen Time Management: Limit exposure to screens before bed to reduce blue light exposure, which can interfere with melatonin production and disrupt sleep.

- **Addressing Underlying Issues**

1. Manage Stress and Anxiety: Incorporate stress management techniques such as mindfulness, meditation, or deep breathing exercises to alleviate anxiety that may impact sleep.

2. Seek Professional Help: If sleep problems persist despite implementing lifestyle changes, consider consulting with a sleep specialist or therapist to address underlying issues and receive targeted treatment.

- **Adapting to Life Changes**

1. Shift Work: For those with irregular work schedules, implement strategies like light therapy, environmental adjustments, and consistent routines to manage shift work-related sleep issues.

2. Travel: Use strategies such as gradual schedule adjustments, proper hydration, and exposure to natural light to overcome jet lag and maintain sleep quality during travel.

Maintaining Sleep Health

- **Regular Monitoring and Reflection**

1. Track Sleep Patterns: Use tools like sleep diaries or wearable trackers to monitor sleep patterns and identify any changes or disruptions. Regularly reviewing this data can help address emerging sleep issues.

2. Reflect on Sleep Quality: Periodically assess your sleep quality and overall well-being. Consider how changes in your routine or environment may be impacting your sleep and make adjustments as needed.

- **Continuous Improvement**

1. Stay Informed: Keep up-to-date with the latest research and recommendations related to sleep health. Staying informed can help you adapt to new findings and incorporate effective practices into your routine.

2. Experiment with Strategies: Be open to trying new techniques and approaches to improve sleep. Individual responses to sleep interventions can vary, so experimenting with different strategies may yield better results.

- **Encouraging Healthy Sleep Habits**

1. Promote Sleep Education: Educate family members and loved ones about the importance of sleep and healthy sleep practices. Fostering a sleep-conscious environment can support collective well-being.

2. Lead by Example: Model good sleep habits and prioritize sleep as a fundamental aspect of self-care. Your commitment to maintaining sleep health can inspire others to adopt similar practices.

Embracing restful nights requires a thorough approach that combines consistent routines, a conducive sleep environment, healthy lifestyle choices, and proactive management of sleep-related challenges. Individuals can achieve lasting improvements in sleep quality and overall health by practicing these strategies. Prioritizing sleep as a vital component of well-being and staying adaptable to changing circumstances ensures that restful nights become a sustainable and integral part of a fulfilling life.